Plastic Surgery Secrets for Breast Augmentation

Answers You Must Have Before Surgery

By: Dr. Susan Lovelle

The Plastic Surgery Review

515 S Main St
Wichita, KS 67202
www.ThePlasticSurgeryReview.com
Copyright © 2013 by Dr. Susan Lovelle

All rights reserved. No part of this book may be copied, transmitted or stored in a database without permission.

DISCLAIMER

This book is not intended as medical advice. It is also not intended to prevent, diagnose, treat or cure disease. Instead the book is intended only to share the unofficial research and opinion of the author. The information is provided for educational purposes only, not as treatment instructions for any disease or ailment. Much of the book is a statement of opinion in areas where the facts are controversial or do not exist. The information in this book should not be considered any more valid than any other type of informal opinion.

The information was not written to replace the advice or care of a qualified health care professional. Be sure to check with your own qualified health care provider before beginning any protocols or procedures discussed in this book, or before stopping or altering any diet, lifestyle, or other therapies previously recommended to you by your health care provider.

The treatments described in this book may have side effects and carry other known and unknown risks and health hazards. The statements in this book have not been evaluated by the United States FDA. Use of the information in this book is at your own risk.

This book is dedicated to Jean Lovelle, whose lifelong journey towards optimal health and wellness —long before it was popular or trendy— earned her the honorary title of Dr. Jean from the many friends and family members she helped.

A Message to All Contemplating Cosmetic Breast Surgery

Whether they are large or small, perky or not, surgically absent or significantly asymmetric, breasts have been intimately associated with women since time began. They can bring life-giving sustenance to newborns, comfort to an older child and seemingly endless fascination to those of the opposite sex.

Because they seem to have become an integral part of what makes a woman female (whether or not this is substantially true —I, for one, don't think it necessarily is), it is no wonder that many women take the next step, wanting to having breasts that are as close to "perfection" as possible. In some cases, whether it is due to trauma, malignancy, or irregularities in growth, there is a real and possibly troubling deviation from the norm, and restoring a more natural form is considered reconstruction.

In many others, though, the choice to make changes in the appearance of one's breasts is just that —one woman's choice. My name is Dr. Susan Lovelle and it is for your benefit and enlightenment that I've written this book.

As a plastic surgeon, I have spent countless hours speaking to women about the various pros and cons of cosmetic breast surgery, the different options available and the right procedure to obtain the results desired. Just as every patient and every breast is different from the next, the proper procedure will likely be different as well. It is daunting indeed to try to explain to the 5' tall, 100 pound woman that she will not get the same beautiful results from the 450 cc implants that her taller and heavier friend received. Nor, in another instance, will putting implants into breasts that are already sagging make them any less so. It has, for many years, been my pleasure to experience the look of joy on a woman's face when the right procedure and the right implant come together to create the perfect look for her. If you are among those who want to experience this for yourself, then ThePlasticSurgeryReviews.com/sign-up and achieve the perfect look you desire.

While I can't condense all of the experience and knowledge I have culled over the years into a book of this size, what I do hope is that many of the questions you have about your upcoming cosmetic breast surgery will be answered in a way that you find valuable. I would love to hear from you as you begin your journey towards having the breasts you have always desired. For all your inquiries on cosmetic breast surgery and anything else that's closely related, feel free to send me an email.

All the best,

Susan Lovelle, MD, MACM
drsusanlovelle@theplasticsurgeryreview.com

TABLE OF CONTENTS

A Message to All Contemplating Cosmetic Breast Surgery 5
CHAPTER 1 – Why Breast Surgery? 8
    What's the Difference Between Cosmetic and Reconstructive Breast Surgery? 8
Chapter 2 – Types of Cosmetic Breast Surgery 13
    Breast Augmentation 13
    Breast Lift 16
    Mastopexy with Breast Augmentation 19
    Types of Breast Implants 21
    Size, Shape and Texture 23
    Anatomically Shaped Silicone-Filled Breast Implants 24
Chapter 3 – What To Expect 26
    Diagnostics 26
    Anesthesia 26
    Dealing with Risks 30
    Who is NOT a Good Candidate for Cosmetic Breast Surgeries? . 31
    Average Hospital Stay 32
    Postoperative Care 33
    What About Post-Surgical Pain? 34
    Will I Have Scars? 35
    Resuming Normal Activity 35
    What About Diet? 36
    What Is Happening to My Breasts? 36
    What About Implant Rupture? 38
    What About Later Breastfeeding? 39
    When to Notify the Doctor… 40
Chapter 4 – Commonly Asked Questions & FAQs 41
    Commonly Asked Questions Regarding Breast Augmentation 42
Chapter 5 – Choosing a Plastic Surgeon 48
    Questions to Ask your Plastic Surgeon 49
Conclusion 51
Recommended Reading 52
About The Author 54

CHAPTER 1 – WHY BREAST SURGERY?

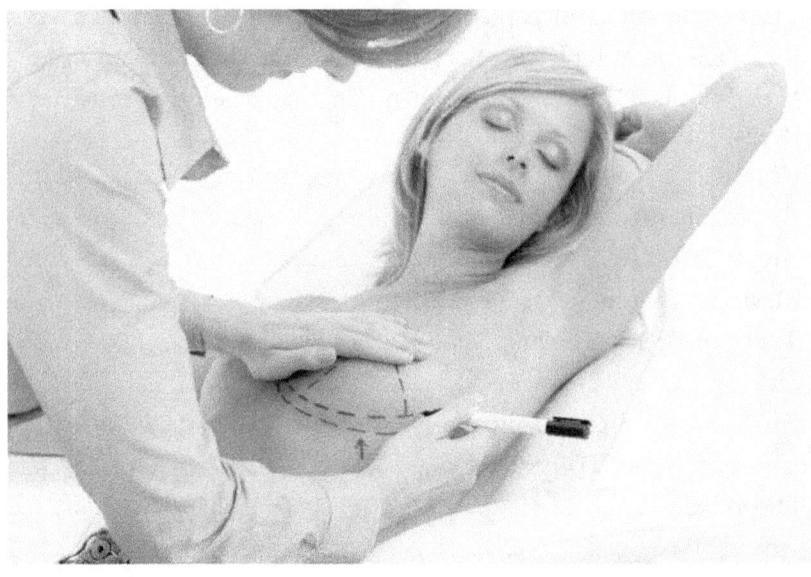

For a number of reasons, many of us are not happy with the shape, appearance, or size of our breasts. Breast surgery provides women with a number of options that help restore balance or symmetry, improve appearance, and change size.

Whether you're looking for breast augmentation, a breast lift, or a combination of the two, cosmetic breast surgery can help enhance your sense of self-esteem and self-confidence.

WHAT'S THE DIFFERENCE BETWEEN COSMETIC AND RECONSTRUCTIVE BREAST SURGERY?

Cosmetic breast surgery and reconstructive breast surgery are different in many aspects. Both are approached for a variety of reasons, but both breast surgery categories are important when facing certain issues regarding your breasts.

CHAPTER 1 – Why Breast Surgery?

In most cases, reconstructive breast surgery is an approach designed to repair an otherwise "abnormal" or traumatized part of body tissue; in other words, issues with form or function. Reconstructive surgeries mainly focus on developmental abnormalities, tissue damage caused by infection, birth defects, the result of trauma, or as a result of tumors or disease processes.

Cosmetic breast surgery is most often a voluntary decision, not made due to deformities, but rather to change or improve the appearance of the breasts. Cosmetic surgery, at its most basic definition, modifies your breasts to enhance a sense of self-confidence and self-esteem based on your perceptions and goals.

Keep in mind that because cosmetic surgery is an elective procedure and does not aid in function or capability in regard to use, it is not typically covered by health insurance policies.

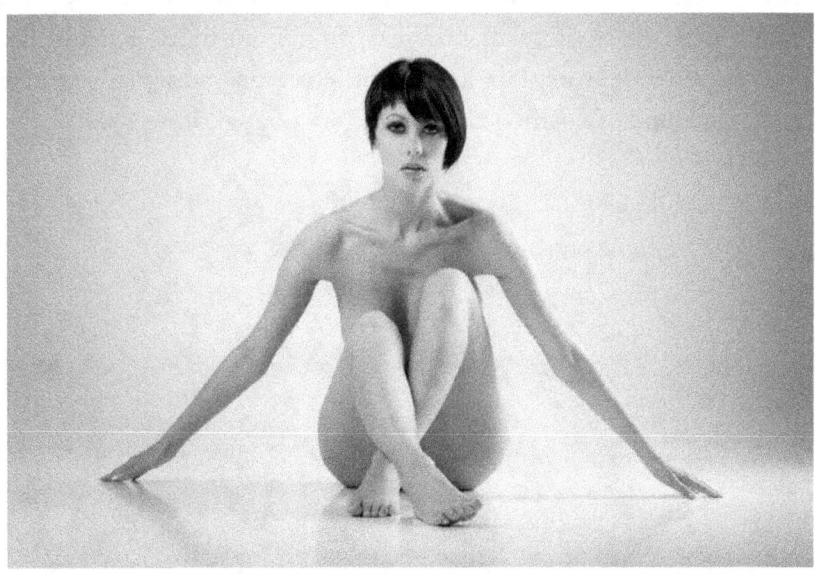

In some cases, procedures such as breast augmentation that are usually considered cosmetic can fall into the reconstructive breast surgery category. This is true especially in the case where the breast

Plastic Surgery Secrets for Breast Augmentation

augmentation is sought in order to reconstruct or improve the appearance of breasts following tumor removal, partial mastectomy, or other traumas. Also, if after reconstructing one breast post-mastectomy the opposite breast is significantly smaller or "droopier," breast augmentation or lift is considered part of the reconstruction and is thus covered by the patient's insurance.

The key to differentiating the two is to remember that cosmetic breast surgeries are not designed to restore form or function, but to alter the shape or size of your breasts. If a surgical procedure is not designed to restore one of the above, it will likely be classified as a cosmetic surgery.

The most common types of cosmetic breast surgery include breast augmentation, breast lift, and augmentation mastopexy (breast lift plus implant). Each of the above use a variety of techniques and many use one of the several types of implants available. We'll explain each of these types of cosmetic breast surgery in more detail in Part 2, but for now, let's explore a few of the reasons why many women choose one type of cosmetic breast surgery over another.

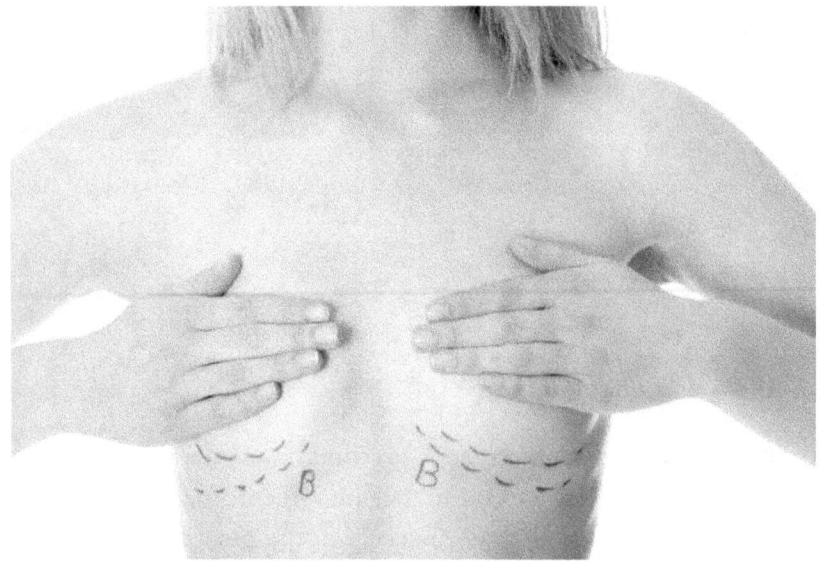

CHAPTER 1 – Why Breast Surgery?

Breast Augmentation

Is a cosmetic procedure that enhances or augments the size of the breast. This is done with either silicone gel or saline implants. In most cases, a breast augmentation procedure is performed to increase a woman's breast size by one or more cup sizes. Many women choose a breast augmentation surgical procedure to increase self-confidence, self-esteem, and improve the proportion or balance of their figures.

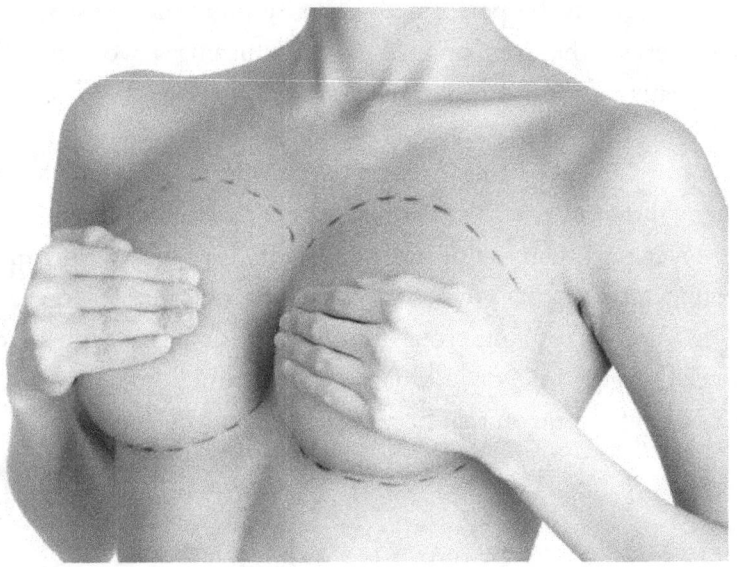

Breast Lift

Also known as mastopexy helps to reshape or raise sagging breasts. Several factors have been implicated in "droopy" breasts: pregnancy, age, and smoking, higher initial cup size, higher body weight, and family genetics. Surprisingly, though, breastfeeding is not on this list; instead, the skin of breastfeeding women tends to be of better texture than those who do not breastfeed although their areolae are larger. Breast lifts usually incorporate some degree of areolar reduction as part of the procedure, making the breast more aesthetically pleasing.

Plastic Surgery Secrets for Breast Augmentation

Aging processes can cause a gradual loss of volume, especially for smaller-breasted women, and a breast lift not only increases firmness and the apparent size of the breasts, but can also be performed at any age. Even women with larger or fuller breasts can undergo a breast lift procedure; although they may be more likely to have sagging recur due the physics of gravity.

When a woman's breasts are both smaller and more droopy than she would like, a combination procedure called an augmentation mastopexy can be performed. This results in a breast that is larger and perkier than the original, often returning a woman to her pre-pregnancy, youthful appearance.

As you can see, breast surgery is an option for many women, for many different reasons. The size of her breasts is extremely personal to every woman, and it's important for every woman to feel comfortable in her own skin. Deciding on breast surgery requires consideration of numerous factors, including the type of cosmetic breast surgery to choose, what to expect, and how to choose a plastic or cosmetic surgeon that best meets your needs and goals.

Chapter 2 – Types of Cosmetic Breast Surgery

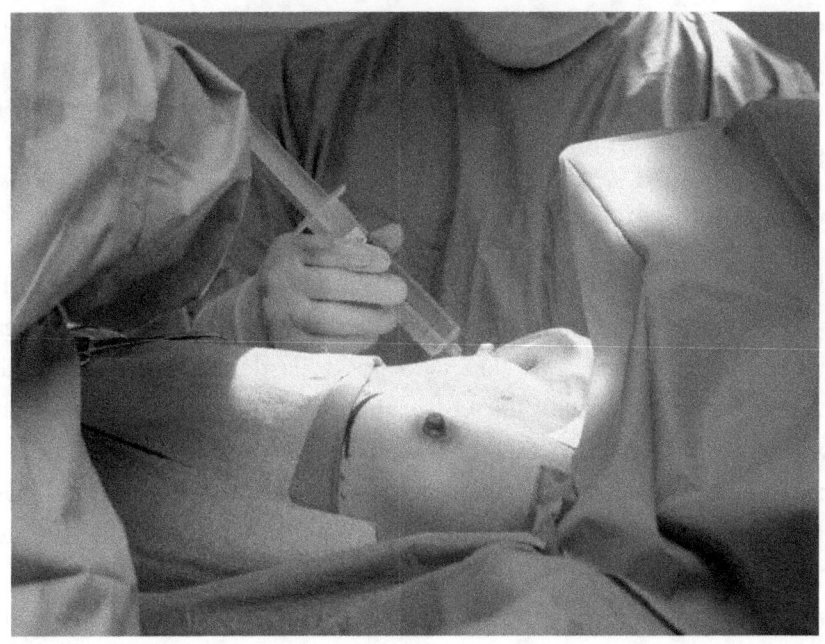

Numerous types of cosmetic breast surgery are available, based on personal goals and needs. From breast augmentation to breast implants, this section will discuss some of the most common types of requested cosmetic breast surgery.

Breast Augmentation

Many women, for a variety of reasons, seek breast augmentation cosmetic surgery; balancing the figure, increasing fullness, and enhancing self-confidence and self-image are just a few of the reasons many women opt for this procedure. Known medically as augmentation mammoplasty, the procedure utilizes a variety of implements and techniques to either restore or increase breast volume.

A plastic or cosmetic surgeon performs breast augmentation procedures. In most cases, women younger than 18 years of age are discouraged from breast augmentation or enhancement procedures, as their bodies have not yet fully developed. Breast augmentation implants will not impair breast health, but time, weight loss or gain, pregnancy, and even menopause may change the appearance of augmented breasts over time.

Who is the Best Candidate for Breast Augmentation?

The optimal candidate for breast augmentation is a woman with small, symmetric, and well-shaped breasts, good soft tissue cover (more on this later), and skin with good elasticity. That being said, there are far more women who don't fit all of those criteria than women who do. Fortunately, women who have different sized breasts or asymmetric shapes are also appropriate candidates for breast augmentation procedures. This includes women who have one or both breasts that have failed to develop "normally." Plastic surgeons generally recommend that a woman's body be allowed to become fully developed before considering cosmetic breast augmentation procedures —time often corrects multiple breast issues, but you won't know until you stop growing.

Benefits of Breast Augmentation

A woman who desires larger breasts, or who wants to improve the appearance of droopy or asymmetric breasts will benefit from a breast augmentation procedure. In some cases, a plastic surgeon may suggest breast lift in combination or conjunction with breast augmentation for women with severely drooping breasts in order to achieve optimal results.

Breast Augmentation Technique

The most common approach to breast augmentation procedures is the creation of an incision, either under the breast in the crease

Chapter 2 – Types of Cosmetic Breast Surgery

(inframammary), around the areola (periareolar), or in the armpit (transaxillary). The location of these incisions is designed to minimize scarring while still providing safe access to the breast, and your plastic surgeon will discuss such options with you before the surgical procedure.

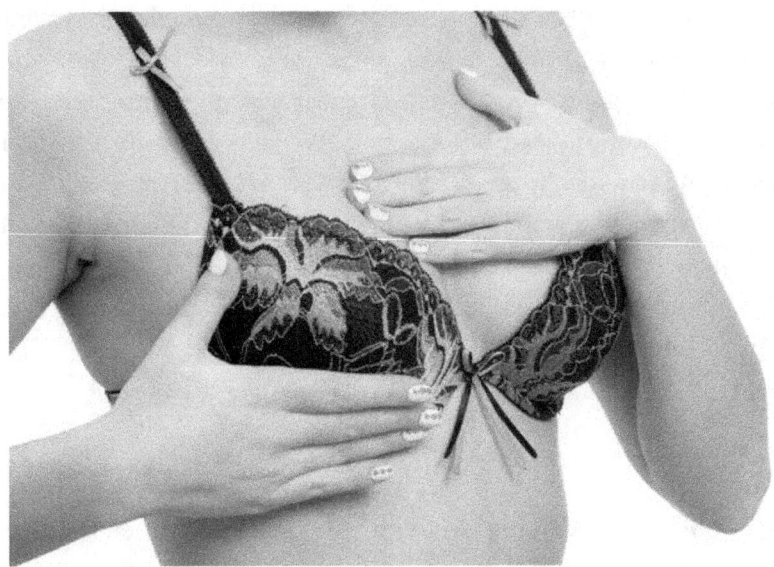

Your doctor will also discuss the two types of implants available —silicone and saline. Saline implants are inserts filled with sterile salt water. Silicone implants are inserts filled with an elastomer type gel.

During the breast augmentation procedure, an incision is made for preparation of the implant. Breast implants can be placed under the pectoral or chest muscle, or immediately behind breast tissue, over the pectoral muscle. The type of implant you have chosen, your body type, and the recommendation of your plastic surgeon will determine the method of insertion and its placement.

The implants are usually soaked in antibiotic solution prior to insertion, and care is taken to handle them as little as possible; this lowers the chance of infection postoperatively as well as other possible complications.

The incision is typically closed with either sutures, a skin adhesive or surgical tape, each of which minimizes scarring. Remember that incision scars will eventually fade over time.

When can I Expect Results?

Results of breast augmentation procedures are immediately visible. However, patients should expect some discomfort, bruising and swelling following the procedure. In most cases, prompt recovery without complications can be expected. Women can return to their normal daily activities after swelling or soreness has resided, most often within one to several weeks following the procedure. Although most patients are cleared to resume full activities - including exercising and running - at six weeks, final results may take several months to achieve.

BREAST LIFT

Many women are dissatisfied with the shape of their breasts, especially when they begin to sag and droop, either after pregnancy or as aging and gravity take their toll on breast tissue, skin, and ligaments. Drooping of the breast is called ptosis, the degree of which is determined by how low the nipple complex sits in relationship to the lower breast crease or inframammary fold. Breast lifts are often recommended to women who experience moderate to severe ptosis.

Chapter 2 – Types of Cosmetic Breast Surgery

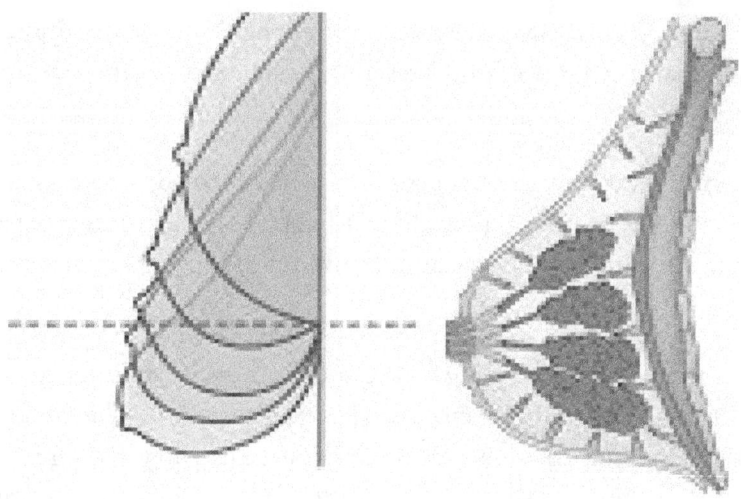

In medical terms, a breast lift is known as mastopexy. It defines a cosmetic procedure that lifts and firms the tissues of the breast, giving them a more youthful and 'perky' appearance. A breast lift procedure usually does this by removing excess skin and elevating the nipple back to its original position; this serves to improve the overall contour and shape of natural breasts.

Breast Lift Techniques

Several breast lift techniques are used today, including concentric or doughnut mastopexy, short scar, and anchor shaped mastopexy. Although each of these techniques utilize a different number of incisions, they are all similar in that the primary goal in each is to elevate the breast tissue and its nipple and areola. Various factors are analyzed to determine the best approach, including skin quality, breast size and shape, severity of sagging or drooping, as well as the location and size of the areola.

When there is minimal drooping of the breast, most lifting procedures concentrate on incisions only around the nipple; the most common is called the donut or concentric mastopexy. In this procedure, concentric circles are drawn around the areola and incisions are made along these circles. Through these incisions, excess skin (and tissue, if needed) is removed. This procedure results in minimal elevation of the breast and can decrease the size of the areola.

It is important that this type of lift to be reserved for breasts with only minimal ptosis as attempting to achieve a significant elevation with this technique may result in significant wrinkling or widening of the areolar border.

When there is more sagging of the breast, there is often more excess skin as well, requiring a more extensive procedure. The other two techniques listed above, short scar and anchor, allow for removal of this excess skin as well as elevating the nipple to its proper position. The incision of the short scar mastopexy is sometimes described as a lollipop as it circles the areola and then drops vertically down to the inframammary fold.

Anchor shaped mastopexy is a procedure generally utilized on larger breasted women, or on women whose breasts have succumbed to gravity, with excessive drooping or sagging; usually the nipple is below the lower breast crease when this approach is chosen. The plastic surgeon may use a pattern to determine how much skin is to be removed as well as the new, elevated location of the nipple areola. The upper part of this anchor drawing is known as the keyhole. It is into this "keyhole" that the nipple is elevated.

To review, the incisions for the three main types of mastopexy include:

- Around the areola.

- Around the areola and downward on a vertical line from the areola to the breast crease.

- Around the areola and on a downward vertical line from the breast crease and horizontally along the breast crease.

During each of these procedures, the excess skin is removed, the nipple is elevated to a more appropriate position, and the remaining skin is pulled up and together. Each of these techniques improves and enhances the appearance of the breast and reduces sagging and drooping.

Depending on the approach, some incisions will be hidden in the breast crease, while others are not. Each technique, location of incisions and potential for scarring should be discussed with the plastic surgeon.

What are the Benefits from a Breast Lift Procedure?

A breast lift procedure helps reduce the appearance of drooping or sagging breasts caused by aging, gravity, weight gain or loss, and pregnancy, as well as hereditary or genetic breast development factors. Breast lift surgery does not change the overall size of the breast, although they may appear to be larger after the procedure. It will give more fullness in the upper portion of the breast, but with the natural slope or pear shape of the youthful breast. For those who wish a more rounded or full upper breast in addition to increased breast size, the next procedure, augmentation mastopexy, may be indicated.

MASTOPEXY WITH BREAST AUGMENTATION

Women with ptosis or drooping breasts who undergo breast augmentation without a breast lift may be dissatisfied with their results. In some cases, a condition known as bulging or 'double bubbles' may occur; in essence, the breast implant sits higher on the chest wall in the original position of the breast while the sagging breast tissue hangs below it, creating a breast with a very artificial and unattractive look.

Breast lifts done at the time of the implantation, known as augmentation mastopexy, place the native breast and the implant in the same elevated position on the chest, making them an integrated, aesthetically pleasing unit.

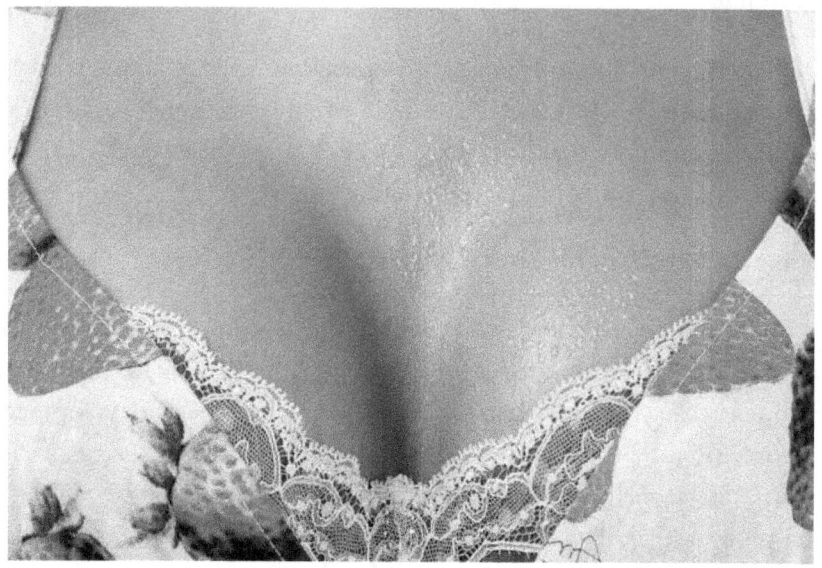

Breast augmentation mastopexy is very popular among women today. As we discussed earlier, while a breast lift naturally increases the appearance of a patient's cup size due to rearranging of the structure of the overall breast, it does not increase the overall size of the breast. For those who desire both a larger as well as a lifted breast, this is an optimal solution. It is also appropriate for those who would prefer a fuller appearance to their upper breast, known as the upper pole.

It is a common misconception that placing implants at the time of mastopexy will lead to perennially "perky" breasts. It is true that implants can provide some much needed fullness of the upper pole to those that have lost that; however, unduly large implants (sometimes placed in a misguided attempt to fill out the excess skin of the sagging breast) will eventually lead to the recurrence of sagging and drooping of the breasts. This may eventually result in a degree of ptosis that surpasses the initial presentation. The implants will, however, preserve their shape as long as the integrity of the implant shell is maintained.

In many cases, breast lift with implants is performed through the same approaches, techniques, or methods as a standard breast lift, although the complexity is increased by the insertion of the implant. Just as in the standard augmentation, the implant may be either saline or silicone, textured or smooth. Similar decision-making with respect to implant shape, texture, or profile as noted above with standard augmentation may be utilized. As mentioned earlier, implants are placed behind the mammary gland or pectoral muscle, giving the patient an immediate change in breast silhouette, shape, and appearance.

Patients undergoing mastopexy with breast augmentation should keep in mind that scars might be noticeable following the procedure. In most cases, scarring is visible from the lower edge or bottom of the areola to the base or crease of the breast. Circular scars around the areola may be visible in women who undergo the doughnut technique for some time. However, in most cases, scarring from surgical incisions fade with time.

TYPES OF BREAST IMPLANTS

Understanding breast implants and procedures is important for anyone considering cosmetic breast surgery. Breast implants have been used for decades, and the materials and techniques for implantation keep getting better and better. While the very first successful breast augmentation may have been with the transfer of a fatty tumor in the late 1890s, it wasn't until the 1960s that the modern day silicon-based breast implant was developed. Until then, various materials such as glass beads, rubber, ivory, and even injections of free silicone had been used unsuccessfully.

In 1961, a Houston physician by the name of Frank Gerow realized while handling a transfusion bag filled with blood, that the texture, firmness, and malleability was a perfect solution for millions of women around the world were dissatisfied with the shape of their breasts. Why Dr. Gerow was thinking about breasts while handling a transfusion bag is unknown, but that year, along with his associate, Dr. Thomas Cronin, Dr. Gerow created the first silicone breast implant.

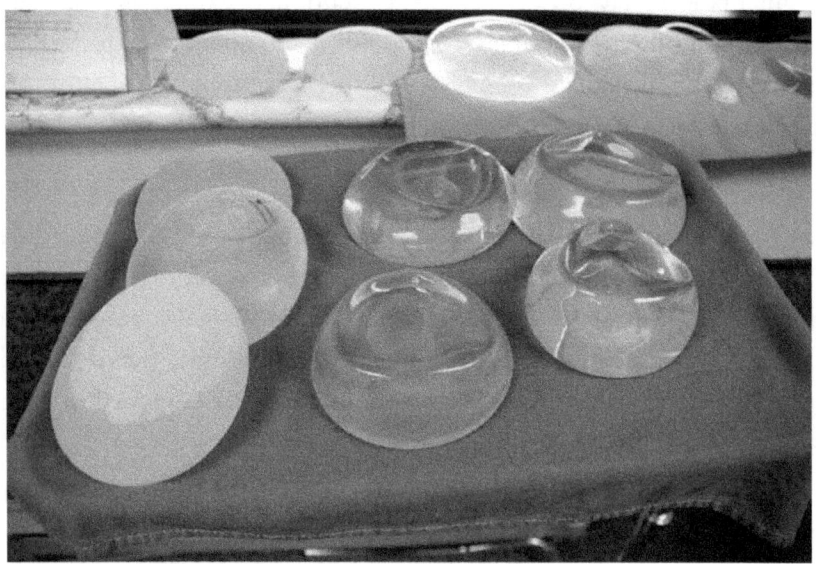

In the 1980s and 90s, claims that breast implants were implicated in both breast cancer and complications in standard augmentations led to the removal of silicone breast implants from the market as well as the bankruptcy proceedings of Dow Corning. Subsequent multinational studies reveal that there was no association with silicone implants in either breast cancer or connective tissue diseases. The one issue with implants at that time was that ruptures of the silicon shell could result in free silicone nodules in the body. Since that time, improvements in both the shell and fill of silicone implants have resulted in devices with an extremely high safety profile.

SIZE, SHAPE AND TEXTURE

The two types of breast implants today, saline and silicone gel, come in a variety of sizes and shapes as well as smooth and textured. Generally, implant sizes range and volume from approximately 120 cc to 850 cc. It's important for you to discuss reasons for desiring breast augmentation as well as your goals before choosing one size or type of implant over another, as not all will result in the shape and proportion that you desire.

Remember that size is not the only factor when choosing a breast implant; your overall body and chest structure will also determine which implant will be most appropriate for you. A woman choosing breast implants that are too large for her frame, and that she can't 'carry' comfortably, may look unnatural, unbalanced, and may even potentially lead to difficulties with posture.

As noted above, in recent years, breast implants have been filled with two popular components -- silicone or saline, a saltwater-type solution. The outside of both types of implants is constructed of an envelope or case called a shell; this is constructed of a sturdy silicone elastomer. This means that technically, whether the implant inserted is gel or saline, they are both silicone products to some extent. That outermost silicone shell contains the filling, either a cohesive gel or saline. As the gel filler is placed by the manufacturer prior to their sale (unlike the saline implants which are filled by the surgeon at the time they are placed in the patient), a patch covers the location of the shell where the filler has been inserted.

Women should keep in mind that implants have a warranty of ten years, and thus, may need to be replaced at approximately that time. This is not to say that if, a decade past insertion, the implants are soft, in good position, and normal on mammography, that they must be exchanged. In addition, unforeseen circumstances such as trauma may necessitate their removal sooner than this.

ANATOMICALLY SHAPED SILICONE-FILLED BREAST IMPLANTS

One of the most common issues with breast implants is their round shape. While many women are more than happy with their new cup size and profile, the symmetrically rounded shape of most breast implants utilized on the market today may make some implants easy to identify. After all, women's breasts have a unique shape, and efforts to design more natural looking breast implants have led to what are called anatomically shaped breast implants.

The anatomically shaped breast implant is designed to look more like a slightly teardrop shape rather than a round shape. One of the most popular is designed and constructed with barrier-shell technology and filled with a silicone gel that is highly cohesive, i.e., more stable in form.

Cohesive silicone gel is softer than highly cohesive silicone gel. This type of breast implant is available in a range of heights and projections (the distance that the implant projects outward from the chest wall).

Because these implants have a preformed shape that remains stable (rather than the regular round gel implants that change depending upon breast shape) these anatomically shaped breast implants are, by necessity, offered in different combinations of volume, shape, height, and projection. This allows for a more personalized choice of breast implant. At present, volume varies from approximately 200 to 650 ml depending on implant shape.

The anatomically shaped breast implant is designed to increase breast size with the quintessentially natural look and is therefore an excellent option for breast augmentation procedures. This type of breast implant is also recommended for reconstruction or revision surgeries as well as to replace breast tissues that have been removed due to trauma, cancer, or breast abnormalities. (Breast implants of this type are not recommended for pregnant women or those who are currently nursing).

Surgical procedures that involve the anatomically shaped breast implant require incisions that are appropriate to accommodate the size, style, and profile of the implant and are typically longer than those made for saline breast implants. In addition, all gel implants, whether the standard round or the anatomically shaped, require a larger incision than saline (which are inserted empty and then filled once in the patient) in order to reduce stress on the implants during their insertion. This minimizes potential for implant deformation as well as gel fractures or fissures during insertion.

Chapter 3 – What To Expect

Whether you're undergoing elective or mandatory surgery, it's important to know what to expect. Regardless of the reason for such surgery, any surgical procedure can be scary for patients. Knowing what to expect helps relieve anxiety, and gives the patient an idea of how to handle pre-operative as well as postoperative care.

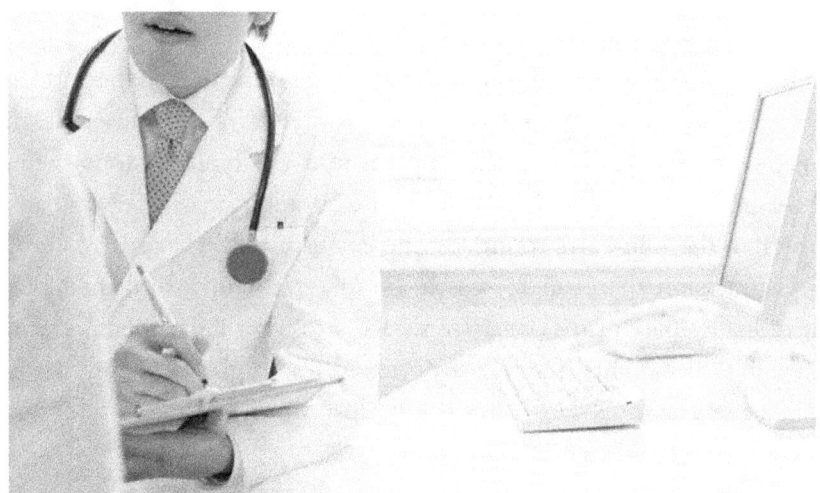

Diagnostics

Prior to any breast surgical procedure, blood tests or studies (and in many cases, a mammogram) will be required. Blood tests will verify that no signs of infection are present (determined by a high white blood count) in a patient prior to surgery. The blood test will also identify any anomalies or abnormalities in blood chemistry levels that may interfere with the safety or efficacy of your surgical procedure.

Anesthesia

Breast augmentation and/or lifts are usually performed under general anesthesia, either through inhalation or injection therapies. In some cases, (for biopsies, for example), local anesthesia with sedation may be offered.

It is extremely important to let your doctor know if you're taking any medication – prescription or over-the-counter, prior to any surgical procedure that requires sedation or anesthesia.

When discussing anesthesia with your doctor or your anesthesiologist, it's important to utilize full disclosure regarding your current health state and medications to your doctor, no matter how minor.

Talk to your doctor about:

- Any previous experience you've had under anesthesia.
- Risks to be aware of, if you smoke or drink alcohol.
- Allergic reactions or any allergies with which you have currently been diagnosed.
- Your medical history, including any prior experiences or adverse reactions to anesthesia, or reactions of other family members to anesthesia.
- Any medications, vitamins, supplements, over-the-counter medications, ointments or creams you may be using.

Keep in mind that prior to use of any type of anesthesia, your doctor may recommend that you not eat or drink for a certain amount of time before your procedure. If you undergo general anesthesia, you are usually cautioned not to eat or drink anything eight to 12 hours prior to the surgery.

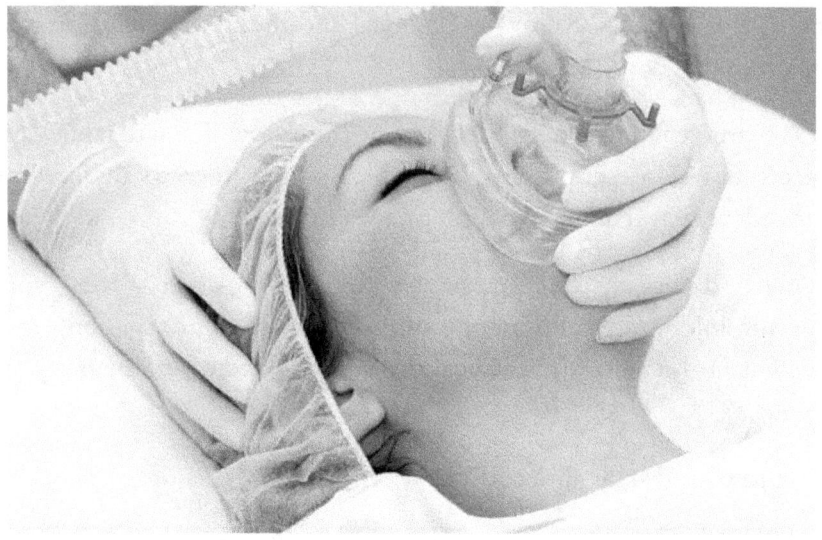

Anesthesia comes in four different types

Local anesthesia - Local anesthesia is often injected into or around the site or area that requires any type of incision, leaving the patient awake and aware. This type of anesthesia may also be applied as a spray or as a topical ointment.

Regional Anesthesia - This type of anesthesia is designed to block nerve signals in a general area of the body. Regional anesthesia is broader in scope than local anesthesia, and can produce relaxation and pain blockage similar to sedation anesthesia.

Sedation - This type of anesthesia is often called "twilight sleep", and is given through an injection intravenously (IV). Sedation anesthesia is often combined with other types of anesthesia during surgical procedures, depending on situation, patient, and length of surgery.

Sedation anesthesia is designed to not only prevent pain, but to reduce anxiety. Twilight sedation is not quite enough to put you into a deep sleep, but can put you in a state of deep relaxation and make you drowsy. Patients are awake, but afterward, don't often recall the procedure. Different levels of sedation are available, so it's important for patients to understand this type of anesthesia, and why it's used in certain procedures.

General Anesthesia - General anesthesia is the type that puts the patient to sleep. The patient is completely asleep and is not exposed to any pain. In most cases, patients placed under general anesthesia don't remember any aspect of the procedure after being wheeled into the operating suite or room. Drugs used in general anesthesia scenarios are either injected through IV into a vein, inhaled, through an oxygen-type mask, or a combination of both.

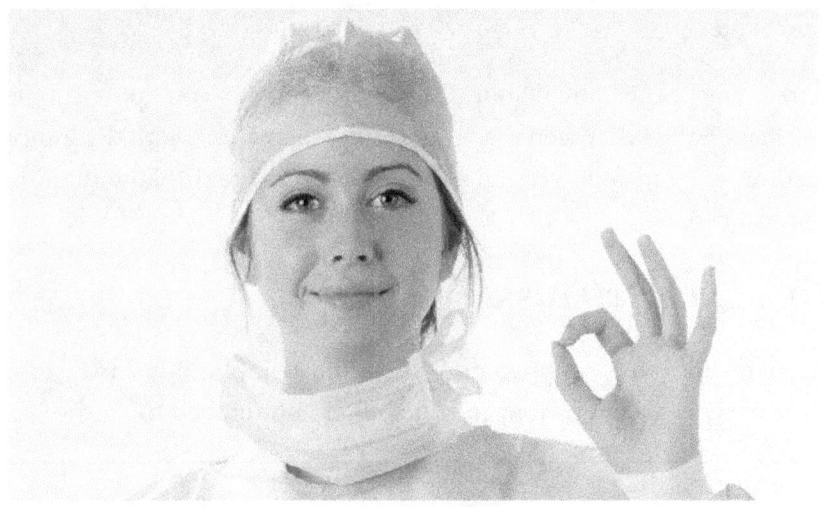

Potential Complications of Anesthesia

Any time an individual receives anesthesia, they are at risk for certain complications or side effects. The most common complication of anesthesia, either with sedation or general, is nausea and/or vomiting. However, perioperative medications today, those administered before, during, or after surgery, are given to prevent such side effects. During many surgical procedures, including cosmetic breast surgeries, equipment in the operating room or surgical suite is in place to monitor blood flow, temperature, heart rate, circulation, and oxygen intake. All of these pieces of equipment reduce risk of complications during procedures.

You will be watched following your surgical procedure to ensure that you are recovering well. During this time, you will be given medications to control your pain and/or nausea if necessary. You will probably have something light to eat prior to being discharged.

Even if you've had a procedure in an outpatient facility, you will be required to have someone drive you home. It is recommended that anyone who has undergone anesthesia have someone who can stay with them or keep them company for 24 hours following the procedure.

After any procedure, your doctor will give you post-surgical instructions and guidelines regarding activity, diet, hydration, medication, and follow-up. Read these carefully and follow them for optimal results.

DEALING WITH RISKS

As with any type of procedure, possible complications may exist. Possible complications may include but are not limited to:

- Infection.

- Excessive bleeding.

- Formation of scar tissue around the implant (this may cause more firmness to the breast than expected).

- Thickened scar or keloid scar formation at the surgical incision site.

- Implants may leak, structure, or become dislodged.

With respect to the above, we are able to take certain precautions prior to, during, and after your procedure. We do give a short course of antibiotics and, in combination with strict sterile technique during the procedure, this is usually enough to stay any possibility of infection. We're also very careful not to proceed with an augmentation if you have an active infection at the time of surgery. This could include skin, respiratory, urinary tract, or any other local or systemic infections. The reason for this is that infections present at the time of surgery may seed the implant, later causing capsular contractures or deep infections.

We also inject a medication at the time of surgery to decrease the risk of bleeding. We ask that you stop any blood thinners such as aspirin or nonsteroidal anti-inflammatory medications such as ibuprofen at least one week prior to your surgery. For those who are on medically necessary blood thinners such as Coumadin, we will work with you and your primary care physician to achieve your goals with the utmost safety.

Although it is not common to develop hypertrophic or keloid scarring with breast augmentation, should this occur, topical medications including steroid tapes or gels usually suffice. Rarely, a formal revision of the scar may be necessary.

WHO IS NOT A GOOD CANDIDATE FOR COSMETIC BREAST SURGERIES?

Breast surgeries, including breast augmentation procedures, may not be appropriate for certain patients.

Relative contraindications or precautions regarding cosmetic surgical procedures include but are not limited to:

- Individuals diagnosed with an autoimmune disease (may include but is not limited to lupus, fibromyalgia, hepatitis, multiple sclerosis, myasthenia gravis, etc.) Talk to your doctor about any prior or existing conditions.

- Women who are expected to undergo chemotherapy or radiation procedures following placement of breast implants.

- Any woman diagnosed with a condition or taking medication that may interfere with or reduce blood clotting and wound healing.

- Any woman diagnosed with reduced blood supply to breast tissues.

- Women diagnosed with a clinical diagnosis of depression, or other mental health disorders, eating disorders, or body dysmorphic disorders.

- Women who smoke must be warned that smoking may inhibit or interfere with healing processes.

AVERAGE HOSPITAL STAY

For most breast surgery patients, again depending on procedure performed, the average hospital stay ranges between an outpatient procedure, where you are released from the hospital the same day as the surgical procedure, to one to two days in a hospital environment. Probable outcomes for breast surgical procedures anticipate complete healing without complication within four to six weeks of the surgical procedure.

Chapter 3 – What To Expect

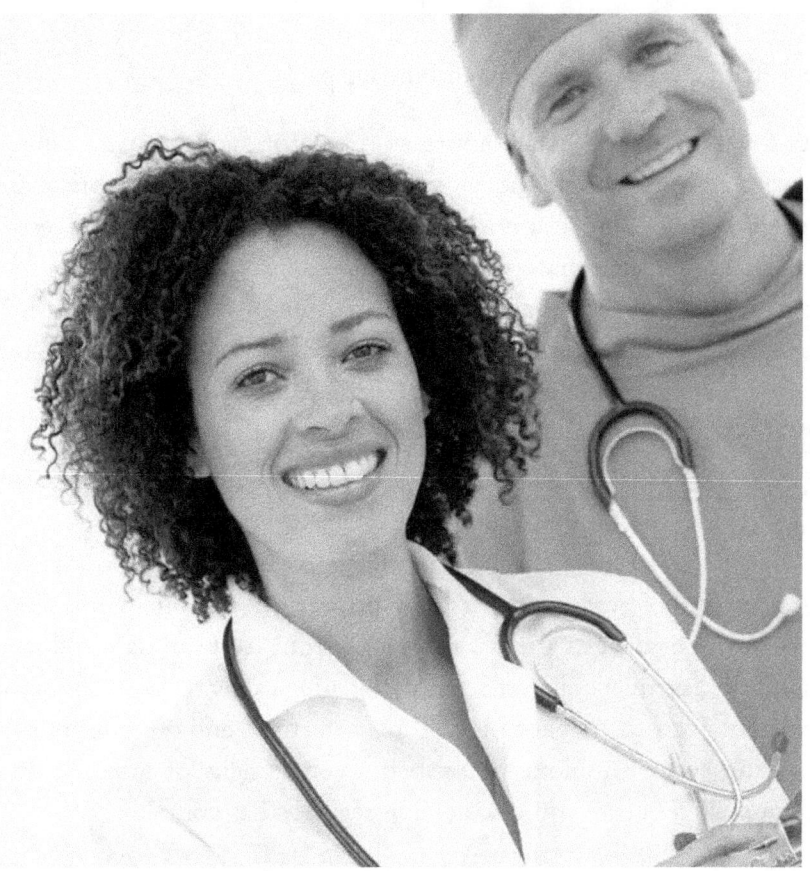

POSTOPERATIVE CARE

General measures for postoperative care apply for most types of breast surgery, but always talk to your doctor and surgeon regarding care of not only the incision site, but also overall health and wellness issues.

In most cases, following surgery you will be able to shower as usual after 48 hours, although you will be advised to gently wash the incision site with an unscented and mild soap.

You can use an ice pack to relieve pain around the incision site as well as to reduce swelling. However, avoid use of ice packs for more than 10 minutes at a time, and protect the skin by placing a washcloth between the skin and the ice pack.

You will be placed in a compression bra for support at the time of surgery; you will continue to wear this (or another appropriate bra) until a follow-up exam determines that he healing process is complete. This may vary depending upon the actual surgery performed, but the usual time frame is four to six weeks. Wearing a bra helps manage the normal post-operative swelling and in some cases, may even help to shape the breast in the early postop period.

WHAT ABOUT POST-SURGICAL PAIN?

When it comes to pain medications or antibiotics, your doctor will advise. In most cases, doctors may prescribe a narcotic pain reliever, but advise against its use for more than four to seven days following surgery. Carefully adhere to instructions regarding its use. Antibiotics will be given to prevent or fight an infection, and it's important to use the entire antibiotic prescribed, even if signs of infection have disappeared before your medication regimen has completed.

Chapter 3 – What To Expect

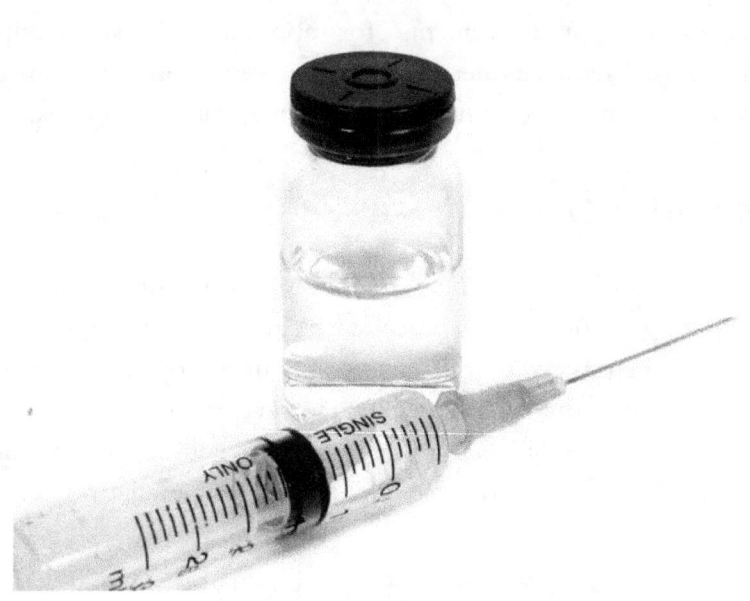

Patients may also take over-the-counter nonprescription pain relieving medications such as acetaminophen for minor pain, although the use of aspirin, ibuprofen, or naproxen should be avoided in the initial healing period. Some people are especially sensitive to aspirin, and it, as well as the others, may also cause thinning of the blood.

WILL I HAVE SCARS?

As mentioned in the description of surgical procedures, you are likely to have some scarring. Depending on the approach as we discussed above, some scars are longer than others. Most scars fade over time, and are barely visible.

RESUMING NORMAL ACTIVITY

In regard to resumption of normal daily activities, your doctor will suggest that you resume your work and daily activities as soon as you feel able. However, you will be cautioned to avoid strenuous or vigorous exercise or movements for approximately six weeks following most breast augmentation, lift or reduction procedures. Most women are able to resume driving activities within one week.

WHAT ABOUT DIET?

There is no special diet you need to follow, except for the day or days leading up to the surgical procedure. Your doctor will give you guidelines on what to avoid prior to surgery, but postoperatively, you may resume your normal dietary habits. However, if you're taking an antibiotic or prescription pain reliever, talk to your doctor about contraindications or foods to avoid while taking such medications.

WHAT IS HAPPENING TO MY BREASTS?

I'm feeling a hard edge…

Patients who have undergone breast augmentation procedures should be aware that a hard ridge may form along the incision site, and sometimes occurs around the edges of the implant itself. This is known as ***capsular contracture***. This type of scarring or contracture causes firmness around the edge or edges of the implant, which can fuel bumpy, hard, and unnatural. For some women, this capsular constructor also causes discomfort.

Chapter 3 – What To Expect

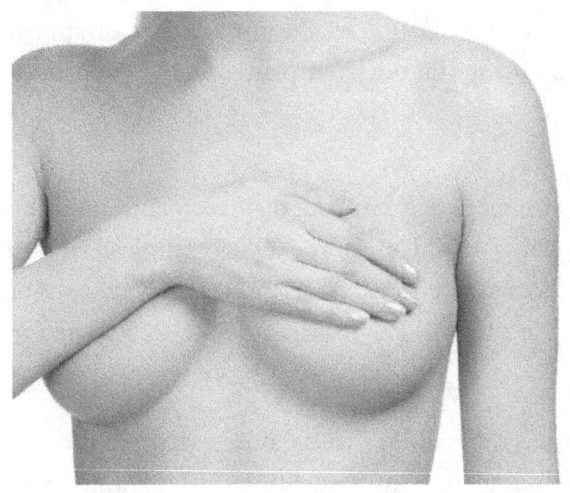

Although older-generation silicone implants had a higher rate of capsular contracture than saline one, more recent studies have suggested that the newer cohesive gel implants may be less likely to develop a significant contracture; it is believed this may be due to the decreased chance of gel leakage. It is important to note that many women may not even notice such contractures. However, in severe cases, the implant may require removal, followed by reinsertion of a new implant. For others, the hardened ridge will heal and gradually fade over time without any additional treatment.

Some capsular contracture scenarios may be avoided by inserting the implant below muscle tissues as there appears to be a slightly higher risk with subglandular (beneath the breast tissue) placement. Textured implants also have a decreased incidence of contracture so, should you choose to place the implants below your breast tissue, it may be advisable to use textured implants in some cases.

My nipples are numb!

Women should be aware that, depending on the type of breast surgery and approach, numbness around the nipple may be noted. Some women may even lose sensation around the nipple area following mastopexy with breast augmentation procedures. In most cases, however, this loss of sensation is temporary and disappears within several weeks following the breast implant surgical procedure.

Oops... I've shifted!

Some women may also experience implant displacement, and while not common, the implants could, in some cases, readjust or drift beneath breast tissues. Women choosing larger size implants should also be aware that they are more likely to drift down, due to gravity, as your body ages.

Talk to your doctor about other things to be aware of when it comes to breast implants, including rippling and implant deflation. In the case of rippling, a breast implant may, after insertion, appear to be wrinkled, or rippled. These wrinkles or ripples are more likely in saline implants and are most often more palpable than visible. The thinner the breast tissue overlying the implants however, the more likely the rippling is to be visible. Smooth gel implants placed under the muscle are the least likely to be affected by this phenomenon. While overfilling saline implants can temporarily decrease the appearance and feel of rippling, it is quite common for some degree of rippling to be present.

WHAT ABOUT IMPLANT RUPTURE?

Many women also ask about the chance for implant rupture. As breast implants are not considered lifetime devices, studies have been performed to determine the incidence of implant rupture. In most cases, very few ruptures of implants occur within the first two years. One implant manufacturer reports a 3-5% rupture rate at three years postoperative and 7-10% at ten years. The rates also differ slightly for saline vs. silicone implants and whether the augmentation was the primary, the first, or secondary.

Chapter 3 – What To Expect

Ruptured saline implants are usually easy to detect: the affected breast fairly rapidly has a deflated appearance when compared to the other breast. Ruptures of silicone cohesive gel implants are not as easy to detect as the gel does not migrate and may well remain within the implant capsule. For this reason, it has been suggested that women with gel implants have an MRI within several years post-procedure and routinely thereafter to determine if there is a silent rupture. In either case, saline or silicone, ruptured implants should be removed, with replacement as the patient desires.

Women should also be aware that since implants are not designed to last a lifetime, removal or replacement will be recommended over the course of their life. Women should also be aware that in the case where implants are removed without replacement, procedures to lift the breast or remove the excess skin may be desired.

WHAT ABOUT LATER BREASTFEEDING?

Women who receive breast implants also need to be aware that their ability to breastfeed may be reduced due to the presence of an implant, either through the reduction or elimination of the ability to produce milk. Areolar and peri-areolar surgical approaches may increase the chance of breast feeding difficulties. Many women have, however, nursed without difficulty after placement of implants. Talk to your doctor about these issues before you decide on approach, implant type, and size.

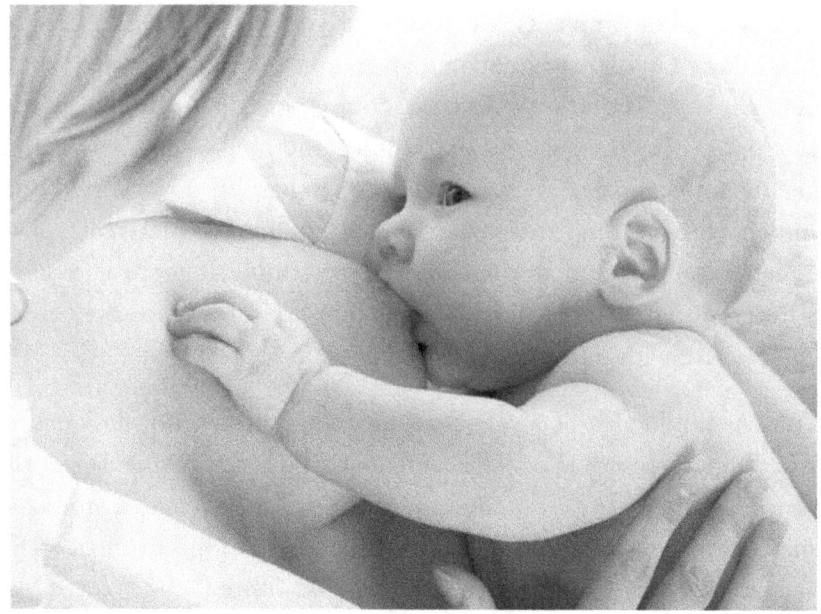

WHEN TO NOTIFY THE DOCTOR...

Be aware of any potential signs that surgical incisions are not healing properly. Always call your doctor if you experience moderate swelling, redness, or pain in the area.

Always let your doctor know if you have continued bleeding or drainage at the surgical site.

Watch for signs of infection which may include but are not limited to muscle aches, headache, fever, dizziness, or a general blasé or feeling of malaise.

Let your doctor know if you have any prolonged or recurring incidents of nausea or vomiting.

Lastly, let your doctor know if you have any of the above, or new or unexplained symptoms following the surgical procedure, as well as those that may be caused by postoperative medications, as some drugs given for antibiotic or pain relief may cause additional side effects.

Chapter 4 – Commonly Asked Questions & FAQs

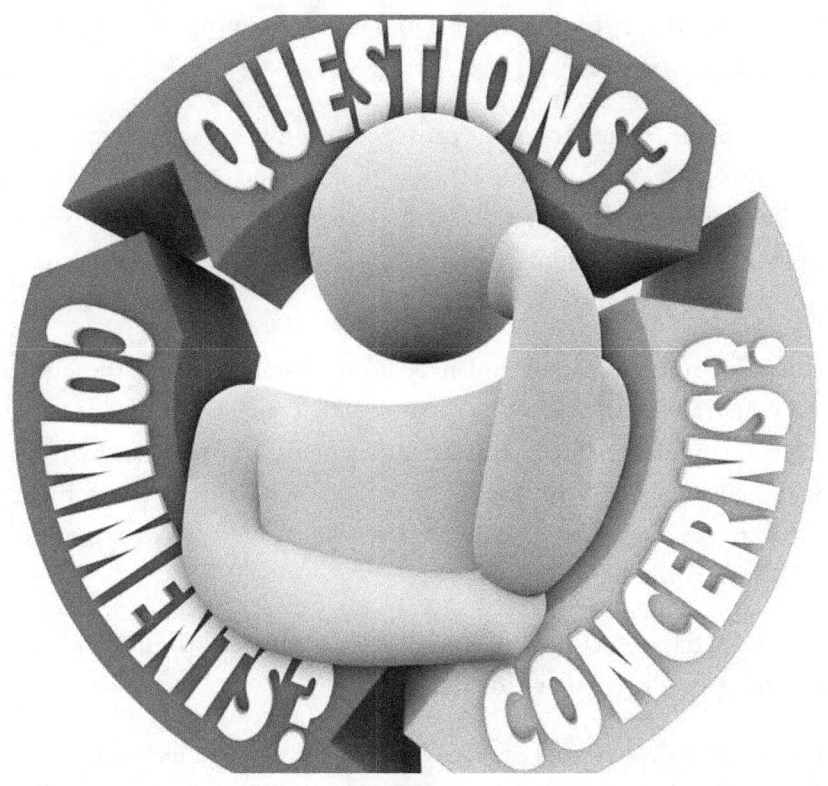

It's normal to have lots of questions to ask about specific cosmetic breast surgeries, as well as questions for your plastic surgeon as well. Don't hesitate to talk to your doctor, plastic surgeon or facility regarding your queries. If you're not happy with the responses or answers you get, take the time to explore your options.

If any doctor or facility hesitates to answer your questions, or brushes them off, it's time to find a different doctor. They may have heard these questions hundreds of times before, but you deserve answers to your concerns and issues.

COMMONLY ASKED QUESTIONS REGARDING BREAST AUGMENTATION

How long do implants last? Do I have to replace them when the warranty is over?

The implant manufacturers provide a ten-year warranty against structural defects, and will replace them at no charge if they fail during that period. They also will cover some of the cost towards replacing them depending upon whether or not you have purchased an enhanced warranty.

This does not mean that you need to exchange them at the end of ten years if you are having no issues with your implants, but rather acts as a guideline for possible replacement. For instance, if you have had your implants for 12 years and have a problem with one implant requiring replacement, I often suggest you exchange them both at the same time.

What is capsular contracture? What causes them and can anything be done to avoid them?

The body naturally makes a covering of collagen (like scar tissue) around anything foreign in the body, including implants. This covering is usually soft and flexible —you don't see it, and you don't feel it. Sometimes, however, the tissue becomes firm for some reason —it is believed that low grade infection may play a factor, although this is not completely clear.

Other causes may be injury to the implant leading to leakage or rupture or bleeding into the capsule. For whatever reason, this hardening of the capsule initially presents as a breast that is firmer than the other but still looks normal. If this continues, the capsule begins to constrict, so that eventually the breast looks smaller and usually rounder and higher than the unaffected breast. In late stages,

Chapter 4 – Commonly Asked Questions & FAQs

this constriction, or contracture, becomes painful and the breast can appear to have a deformity.

Certain steps taken during the actual implantation may decrease the possibility of capsular contracture: placing the implant under the chest wall muscle, using a "minimal touch" technique, use of textured implants, and irrigation with antibiotic solutions. If, despite all precautions, a significant capsular contracture results, the solution is usually surgical —removing the implant and capsule, followed, often, by replacement of the implant. Less severe contractures may be treated non-surgically with medications or external ultrasound.

How soon can I go back to work?

This depends on the type of work you do. Minimally, I suggest taking one week from work if possible. Then, if you have a sedentary job that does not require much upper body and arm activity, you should be able to return the following week.

If your position requires a great deal of arm movement or strength, you may wish to take additional time or have someone help you on the job when you initially return. We will provide a note, if necessary, detailing your restrictions upon returning to work.

How soon before I can go back to exercise?

Lower body exercise, such as walking at a mild pace, can be resumed as soon as you recover from anesthesia. For upper body and more strenuous exercise —running, aerobics, etc., four to six weeks is appropriate. Returning to exercise too soon can slow healing by causing more swelling and sometimes even bleeding.

How long should I wear a bra and what type should I wear?

Although we will place you in an appropriate bra at the time of surgery, you will probably want to obtain a few more before your swelling has completely resolved. An inexpensive cotton bra without underwire and with good support is the best option for early healing. Once you have healed, though, the sky's the limit —enjoy!

What is the best implant for me? What is the best size?

As we discussed in the eBook, there are several different styles of breast implants, and the best fit will depend upon your body type and the final look you want to achieve. The best way to determine your optimal implant style and size is to have a consultation and sizing with your plastic surgeon.

What about mammography?

Today's digital mammography machines make it easier to obtain good quality films with less risk to your implants. Always let your mammographer know that you do have implants; there are some specific techniques they will employ to get the safest, most accurate picture possible.

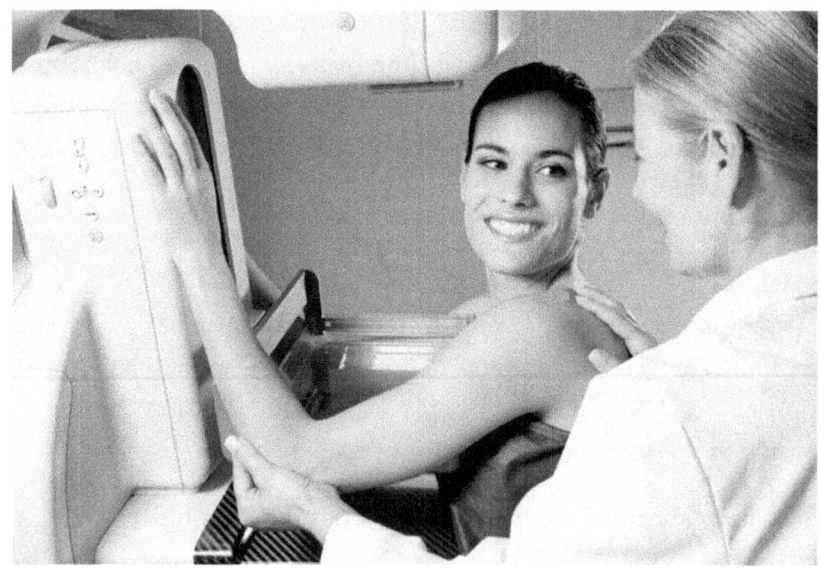

Can I breast feed after augmentation?

Breast feeding is usually possible after augmentation; although some incisions are more likely to be trouble-free than others. Speak with your plastic surgeon if you are definitely planning on having children post procedure.

What if I don't like the size? What if they're too small or too big?

For minor changes in breast size with saline implants, your plastic surgeon may be able to add or remove volume; this would require another surgery to access the fill port. For silicone implants and for larger changes in saline ones, a change in size means the implants need to be removed and replaced. Additional procedures such as a breast lift may be necessary as well.

Am I a good candidate for cosmetic breast surgery?

For many women, this is an extremely personal decision. Consult with the plastic surgeon of your choice and discuss what you wish to change about your breasts as well as your expectations or goals following this cosmetic breast procedure. By understanding all of these, your doctor will be able to provide you with the best options for optimal success and satisfaction.

How soon will people notice a change in my appearance?

When it comes to cosmetic breast surgeries, visible changes are often immediate area depending on the procedure, and whether it's in augmentation, a lift, or a reduction, your appearance or silhouette will change immediately. Subtle changes continue over the first few months, with the final results usually being seen at about three months. Remember that any alteration of your appearance should enhance self-esteem and self-confidence, and not make you self-conscious.

What about recovery time?

Recovery time varies, again depending on procedure. In most cases, women heal quickly, and can recover from a cosmetic breast surgical procedure within four to six weeks. Keep in mind that restrictions regarding physical or work-related activities may be longer, depending on your level of soreness, the procedure, your overall health, and your doctor's recommendations.

For example, a breast implant procedure may take longer to heal than a breast lift procedure alone. In addition, the amount of swelling and bruising experienced post surgically also depends on the procedure as well as the individual. Try not to make comparisons with your friends and relatives who have had similar surgery —your recovery, just as your body, your desires, and your surgery— are uniquely you.

What is the difference between a plastic and a cosmetic surgeon?

Plastic surgery encompasses a number of subspecialties that include but are not limited to cosmetic surgery and reconstructive surgery. In the United States and Canada, cosmetic, reconstructive and plastic surgeons must undergo adequate medical training, most typically composed of four years of medical school, followed by approximately five or more years of plastic surgery preparation and specialty training.

When seeking a cosmetic surgeon, verify that he or she is certified by medical associations or associations in the United States, Canada, or country of residence.

Where do cosmetic breast surgeries take place?

That depends on the procedure. In most cases, consultations will take place at the plastic surgeon's office. Depending on the size of the practice, surgery may be done at a private surgical facility, or at a local hospital or outpatient center where the plastic surgeon has surgical privileges. Always take the time to verify that any facility, outpatient clinic, or hospital, is certified and accredited.

Chapter 5 – Choosing a Plastic Surgeon

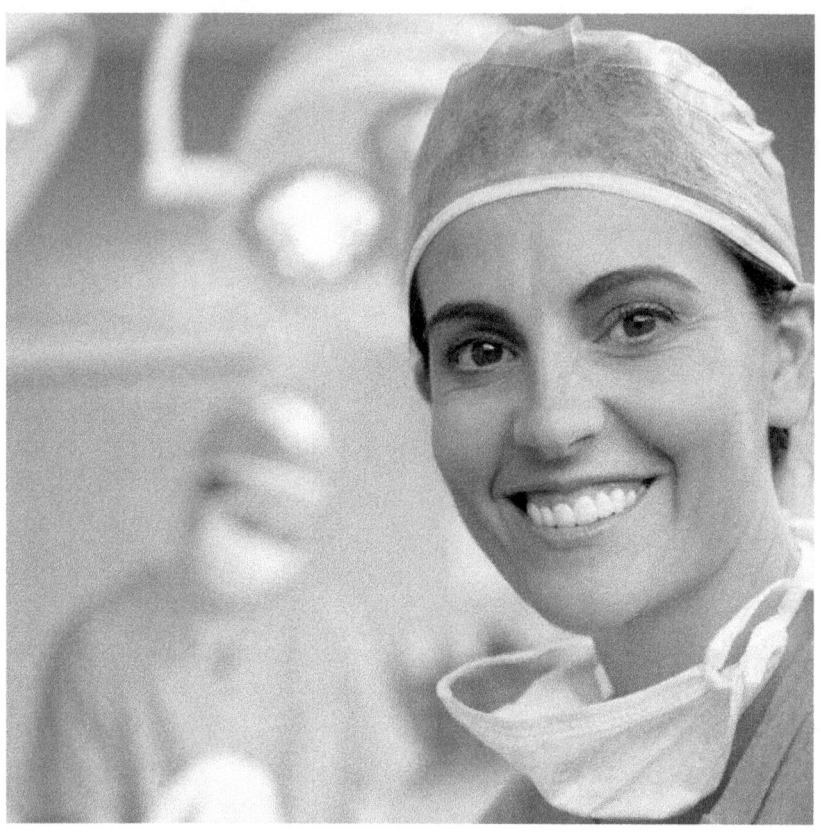

It's important for any woman considering cosmetic surgery, as well as cosmetic breast surgery, to be completely comfortable in the skills, knowledge and experience of her doctor and/or plastic surgeon.

As with the questions about facilities and surgeries, ask questions about your plastic surgeon. A reputable plastic surgeon welcomes such questions and will not hesitate to provide you the answers you seek.

Chapter 5 – Choosing a Plastic Surgeon

QUESTIONS TO ASK YOUR PLASTIC SURGEON

We've covered some commonly asked questions from women seeking cosmetic breast surgery procedures, but will cover several more frequently asked questions not only of plastic surgeons, but about the cosmetic surgery process in general.

When it comes to your choices for a cosmetic breast surgeon, the American Society of Aesthetic Plastic Surgeons recommends that consumers ask a variety of questions about their plastic surgeon. If the plastic surgeon hesitates or refuses to answer such questions, it's time to move on to a new candidate.

Some of the most common questions to ask include:

- Are you certified by the American Board of plastic surgery?
- How many years of experience do you have in (breast augmentation, breast lift, breast mastopexy with augmentation)?
- Did you receive subspecialty training in breast surgical procedures?
- Do you have surgical privileges at the outpatient facility, private surgical suite, or hospital where you recommend I have the surgical procedure?
- If you recommend I have my surgical procedure at a non-hospital based surgical suite or facility, is it accredited by state as well as national accrediting agencies, organizations, or associations?

Don't forget to ask from the surgeon:

- What is expected of the patient in order to obtain optimal results?
- What are the risks of complications or issues that are associated with the specific breast surgery I've agreed to?
- How do you or your office handle issues, complaints, or complications?
- Will I need to deal with implant maintenance or other surgeries at a later point in time?
- What happens if I'm unhappy with outcomes following a breast implant procedure?
- What will happen to the shape and size or appearance of my breasts if I decide at a later point in time to remove the implants?

Conclusion

This eBook has been created to inform and educate women on the most common aspects of cosmetic breast surgery. Of course, you may have additional questions, concerns or issues, and we encourage you to talk to your doctor or plastic surgeon about them.

Cosmetic breast surgery is among the most commonly requested cosmetic surgeries today, and technology, equipment and implantation inserts have advanced by leaps and bounds and continue to do so. Every day, new discoveries are being made, not only in the structure and durability of implants which make procedures safer than ever, but in techniques and types of implants that result in improved outcomes and happy patients.

Make informed decisions, rely on the expertise and experience of your plastic surgeon, and enjoy your new shape to the fullest!

Recommended Reading

The decision to undergo breast surgery for aesthetic reasons is a life changing procedure. One of my utmost concerns is for patients to make educated decisions for themselves on what they really want and knowing what to expect from it. For those who want to learn more on plastic surgery and all that it entails, these are some of the books you will find useful. You can check them out on my site here:

http://theplasticsurgeryreview.com/recommended/

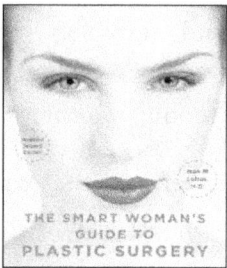

The Smart Woman's Guide to Plastic Surgery, Updated Second Edition

For those considering aesthetic surgery, this book is a must read. From matters such as hidden fees & costs post procedure, to getting the best results from any procedure, this book will definitely prepare you for every aspect concerning plastic surgery.

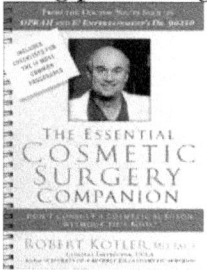

The Essential Cosmetic Surgery Companion: Don't Consult a Cosmetic Surgeon Without This Book!

With all the hype and buzz surrounding cosmetic surgery, it gets quite hard to distinguish factual results from baseless notions. This book provides a clear and concise idea on exactly what to expect from the surgery, what to ask your doctor before the procedure, including the when and where to receive aesthetic surgery.

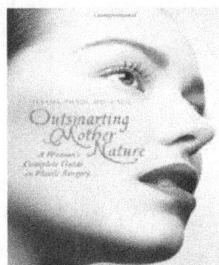

Outsmarting Mother Nature: A Woman's Complete Guide to Plastic Surgery

Get first hand information with all the aesthetic procedures from a female plastic surgeon who not only performs plastic surgery but has gone under the knife as well. With several chapters offering expert opinion and patient point of view, this book will help you tackle the ins and outs of plastic surgery.

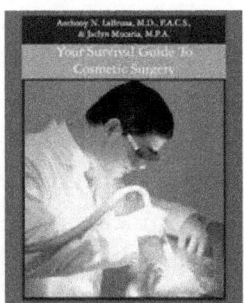

Your Survival Guide To Cosmetic Surgery

Plastic surgery is not as simple as nip/tuck. This book provides a breezy approach in serving as your survival guide through the complex process of cosmetic procedure. From physical preparation to psychological conditioning, this book will help you get ready pre and post surgery.

About The Author

Born and raised in Brooklyn, New York, Dr. Susan Lovelle's artistic talent was discovered at an early age when she was introduced to ballet.

By her teenage years, she had become a principal dancer with the world-renowned Dance Theatre of Harlem, touring in the U.S., Europe, and the Caribbean, and dancing in command performances before royalty in England and Norway.

Although she continued her success as a dancer with the Atlanta and Princeton Ballets, Dr. Lovelle left the world of dance after several years to pursue her childhood dream – medicine.

Medical Background

Dr. Lovelle obtained her medical school training at the prestigious Columbia University College of Physicians and Surgeons in New York City, where she co-authored multiple journal articles on subjects ranging from nutrition to neuroscience. She graduated with numerous honors and awards including Alpha Omega Alpha, the national medical honor society, and the National Medical Fellowship's Franklin C. McClean Award, presented to the most outstanding minority medical student in the nation.

Dr. Lovelle continued her medical training at Columbia-Presbyterian Medical Center where she was one of the first women to complete the rigorous five-year residency program in General Surgery. Propelled by a desire to combine her artistic talents with her surgical expertise, she chose to continue at Montefiore Medical Center where she completed post-graduate training in Plastic Surgery and Microsurgery.

Private Practice

In 1996, Dr. Lovelle began her private practice in Staten Island, New York, where she also founded Armonia, an all-inclusive medical spa facility dedicated to "Health and Beauty through Medicine."

In 1998, her colleagues voted her one of the best plastic surgeons in New York City, an honor highlighted in New York Magazine. As a board-certified plastic surgeon, she was often consulted as a plastic surgery expert by media such as television's UPN 9 on issues such as breast reduction and keloids. She was also one of three physicians chosen to film the pilot for the Lifetime show, "Women Docs" which then became a regular season selection.

Compelled by a desire to practice medicine in an environment that would allow her, both the opportunity for professional satisfaction as well as enjoyment of family life, in 2003, Dr. Lovelle decided to relocate to Elizabeth City, North Carolina, where she owned and operated Carolina Plastic Surgery Specialists. There, she filled a void for both reconstructive and cosmetic plastic surgery, including breast reconstructions, augmentations, and management of skin cancers.

Recently, together with her husband, Board-Certified Ophthalmologist Dr. Kevin Allen, and her two children, the decision was made to accept positions as the first plastic surgeon and the only cataract surgeon based in Newton, Kansas. Drs. Lovelle and Allen, impressed by the commitment of Newton Medical Center to build a regionally-renowned health care system, are pleased and honored by the opportunity to contribute their skills and knowledge to this area.

Drs. Lovelle and Allen are active members of the Newton and Wichita communities – whether sponsoring and participating in fun runs, attending church and leading the youth group, providing vision and skin screenings, or volunteering for civic organizations. Dr. Lovelle was also able to fulfill a long-standing dream when she completed her Master of Arts in Christian Ministry at Friends University in 2011.

You can find Dr. Lovelle on Google+ and Facebook.

www.ingramcontent.com/pod-product-compliance
Lightning Source LLC
Chambersburg PA
CBHW071819170526
45167CB00003B/1368